TESTOSTERONE

BOOST TESTOSTERONE RAPIDLY

The 30 Day Challenge to Transform Your Masculinity

George Aram

TABLE OF CONTENTS

INTRODUCTION

I want to thank you and congratulate you for buying this book, *"Testosterone."*

This book contains a lot of useful information about this hormone, central to masculinity.

Before you start this book, ask yourself these questions:

What do you know about testosterone?

Are you keen to find out about it?

This book will tell you about testosterone and it will explain what testosterone is and how it can be used in a simple yet factual way that does not blind the reader with science. It will tell you about the benefits and the risks of using testosterone.

Most importantly, this book will tell you about boosting your masculinity in 30 days and give hope to those who want to do so.

It will do this without making false promises.

There are 5 chapters, which cover hormones, testosterone, testosterone and age, steroids, means by which testosterone can be given, reality checks, warnings, advice and encouragement. Each chapter will provide a stepping-stone to further exploration, including a 30 day challenge.

CHAPTER 1:
WHAT ARE HORMONES? WHAT IS TESTOSTERONE?

What are hormones?

Hormones are molecules that are messengers that go straight into the blood. This transports them to various parts of the body to execute their functions. These messengers exert control over the majority of important bodily functions, from hunger to reproduction. Hormones have a considerable effect on the moods and emotions you experience. Hormones are manufactured in the endocrine glands of the body. The endocrine glands are ductless hence the direct transmission into the blood. Some major endocrine glands are the pituitary gland which controls other glands (it is often called the master gland), the thyroid gland which controls cell growth, the adrenal gland that controls 'fight or flight' and so on and the list is long.

Some well-known hormones which most people are aware of are adrenaline, the 'fight or flight' hormones, and insulin associated in the minds of most with sugar and diabetes. Other hormones that many people have heard of are cortisol, associated with stress, and melatonin associated with sleep. The hormone we will be focusing on in this book is testosterone usually associated with males. Hormones, which are associated with females, are estrogen and progesterone.

People with hormone problems can have tests, usually by requesting this through their doctor. These tests generally involve testing for hormone irregularities in the blood, saliva or urine.

History of Hormones

The first hormone to be identified was secretin. This was a hormone involved in digestion and was identified in the mid-19th century. There have been many more hormones discovered since then. In order to be identified as a hormone, a chemical has to be released directly into the blood from a ductless endocrine gland and taken to another site in the body by the blood.

What Is Testosterone?

This is regarded as the male sex hormone. Women also have testosterone but in much smaller amounts. In males, a small quantity of testosterone is manufactured in the adrenal glands, which are on top of the kidneys. The most important product of the adrenal glands is adrenaline, which is the 'fight or flight' hormone. The majority, or 95%, of testosterone, is made in the *testes* or *testicles*. All men and most females know that the testicles, often called *balls*, are an appendage on a male body behind the penis.

In actual fact that appendage is called the *scrotum*, a sac of skin, which contains two glands called the testicles or testes. The testes are most interesting organs. They are primarily composed of tubules, which produce sperm; this is the male contribution to sexual intercourse and human reproduction. These tubules have within them testosterone producing cells. In males, testosterone is responsible for the production of sperm and for the development and maintenance of male sexual characteristics. The secretion of testosterone is mainly governed by *gonadotropin* levels in the blood. Gonadotropin refers to a number of hormones.

How Males Use Testosterone

The secretion of testosterone in males carries out the following functions:

(1) It promotes what is generally regarded as *machismo* or *masculinity*, by the development and upkeep of male secondary sexual characteristics, including such organs as the prostate gland, the seminal vesicles and male sexual behavior. It is very closely associated with the male sex drive and has a major role here.

(2) It helps to regulate the metabolism and is sometimes called the *anabolic* hormone as it stimulates protein *anabolism*. This means it helps turn protein into far more complex chemicals. This process is the opposite of *catabolism*, which is the digestive process. In doing this, it promotes the growth of muscles and bones.

(3) It affects the way men store fat in their bodies.

(4) It has a role to play in blood production.

(5) A man's mood is often influenced by his testosterone levels. Testosterone is what drives many men in sport, business, work and life.

The manufacture of testosterone is minimal pre-puberty but increases massively during puberty, and declines after the ages 30 - 35.

How Females Use Testosterone

Testosterone is a sex-related hormone and, as such, plays a role in a woman's sexuality. In females, there are no testes. Testosterone is made in the ovaries, in the fat cells, and in the adrenal glands. Testosterone has many uses in the female body as well as the male. One of those is as an anabolic hormone.

As this book is predominantly for men no more will said about this. There are some very good books on this topic such as *The Secret*

Female Hormone by *Dr. Kathy C. Maupin.* There is also a wealth of material on the Internet although much there is commercially driven.

Steroids, cholesterol, and testosterone

Readers may have heard of steroids. The public perception of them is a performance-enhancing drug taken by many athletes in a variety of sports. In actual fact, steroids are far more than that. They are a very important class of chemicals within our bodies, which have a variety of uses.

Testosterone is a steroid made from cholesterol which itself is a steroid. Cholesterol is another chemical that has a poor public perception. The public is led to believe that cholesterol is the root cause of heart attacks and strokes and that it must be avoided at all costs. In actual fact, cholesterol is a compound found in most body tissues. Cholesterol and its derivatives are very important parts of cell membranes and a forerunner of other steroid compounds.

Three types of testosterone

Most mature men produce around 4-7 mg of testosterone a day. This moves into the blood where it is found in three forms. It is worth noting that the level of testosterone in the blood varies throughout the day. The highest levels are found in the mornings while the lowest levels are in the evenings. There are three types of testosterone in the blood:

(1) The first type is free testosterone, which is not attached to any proteins. Only about 3% of testosterone is free. This sort is the most useful for carrying out testosterone's functions.

(2) The second type is SHBG bound testosterone. This is testosterone that is bound to a protein called SHBG. This testosterone is inactive. It constitutes about 50% of the testosterone in the blood.

(3) The testosterone which is not free or SHBG bound is bound to a protein called *albumin* which is manufactured in the liver. While this testosterone is also inactive it is far more easily used,

as the bonds between the albumin and testosterone are easily broken. This enables testosterone to carry out its functions.

History of testosterone

Like all hormones, testosterone has an interesting history. The connection between masculinity and the testicles has long been known. The use of eunuchs to guard the harems of sultans and emperors is thousands of years old. A eunuch is a male who has had his testicles removed. The reasons that eunuchs were used for guarding harems were that they had no sexual interest in the lovely young ladies who were members of these exclusive organizations.

One of the features of puberty in males is the deepening of the voice. If a male is castrated prior to puberty he retains the light voice he had as a boy and the practice of castrating boys who were good singers was practiced and continued in Italy until the 19th century.

It was during the 19th century - not long after the discovery of the first hormone secretin - that it was established by experiments on roosters that testosterone is a hormone. It was also during this time that the first recorded experiments of testosterone injection were tried.

CHAPTER 2:
TESTOSTERONE AND AGE

Testosterone Levels

Testosterone levels are measured in Nanograms per deciliter (ng/dl). A Nanogram is a very small amount. There are 1000000 Nanograms in 1 milligram. There are 1000 milligrams in a gram. There are 1000 grams in a kilogram and there are 2.2 pounds in a kilogram hence a Nanogram is less than 36 trillionths of an ounce!

A deciliter is one-tenth of a liter. Hence a deciliter is about 3.814 fluid ounces.

Here are some testosterone levels in healthy males.

Age	Testosterone Level (ng/dl)
0-5 months	75-400
6 months-9 years	7-20
12years-13years	7-800
14years	7-1200
17years-18years	300-1200
25years	270-1070
35years	257-1017

40years	243-963
50years	216-856
70years	162-642

There are a few points that need to be emphasized:

(i)   At any age, there is a great range of testosterone levels that are regarded as 'normal'.

(ii)   Testosterone levels are high in the first few months of life.

(iii)   Testosterone levels are low until sometime from about 11 years old until 15 years when puberty sets in.

(iv)   During the late teenage years, testosterone levels are the highest most men ever experience.

(iv)   From ages 20 years - 30 years testosterone levels are pretty constant in the range 270 - 1070.

(v)   After age 30 there is approximately a 1% decrease per year.

Puberty and Adolescence

As can be seen from the table above, the first biochemical indication of puberty in boys is an increased concentration of testosterone in the bloodstream, a phenomenon that generally occurs about a year before the first signs of puberty are perceptible as such to the young person. The first sign of the onset of puberty that is observable to others is the beginning of a period of rapid physical growth called the *growth spurt*. The growth spurt begins with a rapid gain of weight. Towards the end of middle childhood, both boys and girls become heavier, mainly through the buildup of fat, especially on the legs, hips and stomach. Soon after the growth spurt of weight occurs, there is a height spurt, this usually leads to a redistribution of the recent fat. Often during this time, a little boy becomes a pudgy 12-year-old then a lanky 14-year-old, perhaps even taller than one or both of his parents.

During this time, the quest for new experiences is quite usual for boys, and sometimes it shows itself as a desire for thrills, provided by activities such as skateboarding, BMX riding, surfing etc., or even behavior which is, to say the least, risky or illegal. It is quite normal for teenagers to want new experiences, although it can be very trying for you a parent or teacher.

Teenagers have a built-in need to test their own limits and abilities as well as any boundaries set by parents or school. They also need to express themselves as individuals. It is a vital part of their route to development as a functioning, independent young adult.

Sadly those portions of the brain that are involved in planning and the control of impulses usually become fully mature around the age of 25. For this reason, it is more probable for teenagers, than for adults, to make decisions without thought for the consequences. Another thing that is far more important for teenagers than adults is the great need for peer approval.

For boys, it is desperately important for a significant male, preferably their father but failing that an uncle, grandfather, teacher, coach etc., to guide them through this turbulent time and be their support and guide. Once a young fellow reaches maturity and has started to function as a man then this figure should step back.

Hormonally once a male becomes a mature man then his testosterone levels fall back from the peak during adolescence to about 270-1070 ng/dl. There is great variation between individuals and a man's level depends on the time of measurement.

Testosterone levels are highest in the morning but diminish during the day. There is a period of about ten years though when a man's testosterone levels are fairly constant then at the age of about thirty a reduction begins of about 1% a year. This occurs with the following physical effects.

(1) More difficulty in recovering from physical effort;

(2) More difficulty in getting 'psyched up';

(3) A reduction in physical powers. Men such as Roger Federer and George Foreman are not normal in being able to continue their sporting careers, at the highest level, past 30;

(4) A loss of libido although there are plenty of cases of men in their seventies and older who have fathered children;

(5) Hot flushes;

(6) Lack of confidence.

These effects have not been shown to be caused by fading testosterone but they just occur as the testosterone is diminishing.

The result of these changes sometimes leads to consequences that are quite bizarre. Here are a couple of examples, extreme but very pertinent, of men who seemed to go through a *reverse adolescence*. The experiences of their teenage years were repeated to a certain degree with very hurtful consequences for all concerned.

These two examples are based on real-life examples, both well known to the author. I have changed names and details so that identification would be very difficult. The reason I have done this is the prevention of embarrassment and humiliation for the men involved and their families.

James

In the 1960s I became acquainted with a young man who was a gifted sportsman. He went from achievement to achievement in his chosen sport and actually went to the highest international level. During the time of this increasing prowess in the sport, he was also developing his career and personal life. He probably got married too young. However, this marriage was to a very attractive and intelligent woman, and due to his seemingly boundless energy and ability, he was able to purchase a wonderful home. He also reached a managerial status in a competitive industry.

As he reached his 30s, things start to unravel in his life. His marriage broke up and he moved sideways at least twice into new careers and business ventures. He got married five times in total.

On the fourth occasion when he got married he was into his mid-50s. During the marriage ceremony, his son from the first marriage gave a speech at his father's wedding in which he said,

"Welcome Heidi, it is just like having the younger sister that I never had!" Heidi left him soon after the wedding.

He is now with wife five, a marriage that has so far lasted for 10 years and perhaps he has finally settled down. He is the best example from my own life of men I have known who, to combat their fading testosterone levels, acquire new hobbies, business ventures and wives.

David

Another example of this bizarre behavior comes to mind as I cast my mind back over my own career. I was for many years a high school teacher and at one school I was working with a pupil whose parents I met for the first time when he was about 14. The parents owned a building business and were in their mid-30s. Everything seemed okay except that the husband's fading testosterone levels coincided with his appointment of a new secretary. She was a pretty little blonde who he became completely infatuated with, and he consequently broke up his existing marriage and started a new life.

He soon became a father again with this new wife and the years passed by. His business continued even though his first wife had made sure that she got her share of it. I was at a second school when I met his offspring with the second wife. The boy had the blonde hair and mediocre intellect of his mother. I met the father and the new mother at a meeting of parents and teachers. His father looked like a broken man. The energetic, confident person that I had known 15 years before had ceased to exist and had been replaced by a seriously overweight man with massive health problems. It was a reminder to me of the dangers of men who allow their fading testosterone to influence their choice of lifestyle.

It can be debated ad infinitum as to whether the erratic and hurtful behavior of either of these men was caused by fading testosterone or by other factors. In each case, I saw pathetic attempts to grasp at something that had passed in the hopes that it could be resuscitated.

CHAPTER 3:
STEROIDS AND OTHER PERFORMANCE ENHANCING SUBSTANCES IN SPORT

What Are Steroids?

Steroids were mentioned briefly in Chapter 1 in the section "*Steroids, Cholesterol and Testosterone*." It was pointed out that steroids are a very important class of chemicals within our bodies, which have a variety of uses. It was also mentioned that testosterone is a steroid made from cholesterol which itself is a steroid. In the eye of the public, the word steroids will always be associated with performance enhancement in sport.

Are Steroids The Same As Testosterone?

Testosterone is a steroid but not all steroids are testosterone. Testosterone can be used as a definite performance enhancer in sport but probably with more side effects than some other steroids. This will be discussed in more detail later in this chapter.

Does Steroid Use Enhance Sporting Performance?

It is an incontrovertible fact that steroids increase strength if dedicated sportsmen use them. Most serious athletes who use steroids will gain at least 10% increase in strength, with some gaining far more with gains of up to 50%. In addition, steroids help any athlete recover from their workouts more quickly. For this reason, they are of great use to all athletes, even endurance athletes. It must be stressed that steroids are only of benefit if hard training is occurring. Their use in the absence of this effort is a complete waste of money.

Can Females Use Steroids?

Females can definitely take steroids and in doing so they reap the same anabolic benefits as males. The reasons that females are reported to use steroids include a reason not reported by men. This is the belief that if they take steroids they will be strong enough to repel the attack of a rapist. This has been reported as being particularly prevalent among women who have been raped.

What Are The Negative Effects Of Steroid Use?

Among the problems that some men have as a result of using steroids in excess is irrational aggression (this is called 'road rage'), dreadful acne, the swelling of the testicles, the shrinking of the testicles, the shrinking of the penis, pain or difficulty during urination, a reduced sperm count, liver damage, blood pressure problems, erectile dysfunction and impotence. More seriously some men suffer from something called gynecomastia which is a complaint affecting males where the breasts become enlarged. In some men who have abused steroids, this has included the development of secondary nipples.

The effects on the woman can be even more serious. Not only are they prey to the male problems, except those which are exclusively male, they can have a deepening of the voice, a change in the menstrual cycle, a reduction in the size of the breasts, enlargement of the clitoris and a greatly increased growth of hair on their face. As with men women who abuse steroids have often been known to suffer from a lack of libido. The effect can be a complete loss of femininity. Examples of this can readily be seen on the Internet.

During the time of the Cold War between the Soviet Bloc and the West, there was very widespread, state-sponsored, systematic doping of athletes in most East European countries. The former Communist East Germany took this to an extreme degree with at least one of their top female athletes becoming a man as a result of the masculinizing effects of her doping regime.

What Are Some Well-Known Steroids?

Among the many artificial steroids used widely are Winstrol, Dianabol, Anavar and Deca-Durabolin. The first three are usually orally administered while Deca Durabolin is usually injected. Dianabol was invented in 1957, and has been widely used with great success thereafter. Anavar is not nearly as strong as some other steroids and is recommended for use by women who want the benefits without the horrible side effects. Deca Durabolin has been around for decades since 1962. It is still widely used. **People considering their use need to be aware that possession of them without a doctor's prescription is illegal in many countries, including the USA.**

What Effect Has Testing Had On The Use Of Steroids?

In the mid-1970s and onwards the use of steroids by drug cheats became ever more difficult as a result of testing regimes instituted by most international sporting bodies. There was a switch to pure testosterone as a replacement for the artificial steroids. At that time the use of testosterone could not be detected as it is naturally present in the body. It was only a matter of time before this too could be tested for and so the users of these substances switched to designer steroids, which had never been used before and for which there were no tests. The competition between users and testers is ongoing, particularly as state sponsorship of the use of performance-enhancing drugs is practiced in a number of countries.

What Other Substances than Steroids Boost Sporting Performance?

There are lots of substances, which do this. Among them is human growth hormone, amphetamines, EPO, blood doping etc. It is not the intention of this book to detail how each of these boost performance except to mention their use.

Who Uses Performance Enhancing Drugs in Sport?

It was told to the author that a survey of top athletes included the question, "If there were a completely undetectable drug which guaranteed you an Olympic Gold Medal but would halve the length of your life would you take it?" Astonishingly nearly 50% said they would. Given that mindset and the great financial rewards which success in a sport at the highest level brings it is no wonder that so many great sportspeople have used performance enhancing drugs. Among them are Barry Bonds in baseball, Lance Armstrong in cycling, Ben Johnson in athletics and many more.

Summary

The purpose of this chapter was to show how testosterone and its derivatives can be misused. The remainder of this book will be to illustrate a very positive and wonderful effect of testosterone, which is that it can be used to restore a man's self-esteem in a completely wholesome way.

CHAPTER 4:
HOW TO ADJUST TESTOSTERONE LEVELS

This chapter is written for those who wish to elevate their level of testosterone. It sets out how this can be done, discussing the merits of the different methods. The main reason for increasing testosterone levels is *hypogonadism*. Hypogonadism is defined as a situation where the testes in the male do not produce enough testosterone naturally. It also applies to a situation where the production of sperm cells is deficient however this is not considered. Whether you have hypogonadism can only be confirmed by determination of your testosterone levels which involves blood tests.

How Can Testosterone Levels Be Adjusted?

Testosterone levels can certainly be adjusted. There are a number of ways this can be done. However, before this is done there should be thorough medical testing to ensure your suitability. Self-medication is dangerous! Testosterone can be directly administered with results and methods set out below or the body can be encouraged to produce more testosterone by what are called *testosterone boosters*.

What Is The Result Of Directly Administering Testosterone?

Testosterone levels are falling in the Western world. There have been studies showing this. Many men are taking testosterone artificially. Testosterone is a class C drug, meaning that it is illegal without a medical prescription. There are many promises about the good effects of taking testosterone among these are:

(1)   An increase in strength;

(2)   An increase in muscularity;

(3)   An increase in libido;

(4)   A slowing down of the aging process.

The increases in strength and muscularity are definite facts if you are training hard. You are wasting your time and money if you think you will get strong and muscular just by having testosterone administered without some serious effort. At least half a century of performance enhancement in sports has proved this time and time again.

Libido, however, is something different. Libido is governed by a number of factors and a lack of libido can be blamed on things other than low levels of testosterone. It has been shown, however, that in men with low levels of testosterone, and who also have libido problems, there has been an improvement in their libido when they are given testosterone supplementation.

The slowing down of aging is the most controversial claim. There is no study that has demonstrated that slowing down of aging occurs when testosterone is administered. If this claim had been demonstrated then it would be the most important finding of science ever. Testosterone would be the elixir of life. Sadly no one has ever shown that it, or anything else, is.

Now for the negative effects:

(1)   Acne;

(2)   Fluid retention;

(3) Prostate problems, particularly if the recipient has prostate troubles anyway;

(4) Increased risk of blood clots, particularly for men with cardiovascular problems;

(5) If a man receives testosterone from an external source the natural production of testosterone within him ceases!

This latter is not something to be taken lightly. If the body's own production ceases then an extremely serious problem has arisen.

How Can Testosterone Be Directly Administered?

The testosterone supply can be increased by one of a number of methods of external administration. The most common method is that of injection using a syringe. Other methods by which testosterone can be successfully administered are using creams, gels or patches. It is usually not a good idea to administer testosterone with a pill.

What Is A Testosterone Booster?

A testosterone booster is an herbal supplement whose purpose is to cause your body to produce more testosterone or to inhibit hormones, which cause the body to convert testosterone to estrogen, the female hormone. Among such supplements are d-aspartic acid, tribulis terrestris and some zinc compounds. There are a variety of commercially available products, which include some of these and other compounds. As with all testosterone administration, it is essential to follow medical advice and not to self-medicate if you wish to use testosterone boosters.

Summary

Testosterone supplementation will definitely increase strength and muscularity if you train hard. Improvements in libido have been demonstrated as a result of testosterone use. Increases in longevity resulting from testosterone administration have NOT been shown: -

EVER. There are compounds available which claim to stimulate the body's production of testosterone. Any adjustment of testosterone levels should only be done under medical supervision.

CHAPTER 5:
IS IT POSSIBLE TO TRANSFORM YOUR MASCULINITY IN 30 DAYS USING TESTOSTERONE?

What Is Masculinity?

If you were to ask 100 people to define masculinity you would get many answers but if you have a very close look at these answers and do a lot of research about this you will find that masculinity embraces all the virtues that a warrior in the time of hand to hand combat would have possessed. Virility, courage, enormous strength, great stamina, a superb physique plus a whole lot of ideals which knights belonging to King Arthur's Round Table possessed. It is extremely unlikely that Sir Lancelot was deficient in testosterone.

Can Testosterone Help?

I think that I have demonstrated in this book that testosterone can greatly increase all the physical attributes of masculinity provided any attempt to adjust testosterone levels is accompanied by a lot of very hard work. There is no free lunch. If you are stupid enough to think you can become strong, have great stamina and be built like Mr. Olympia without a lot of hard work then you are likely to see the Easter Bunny and the Tooth Fairy in Santa's sleigh.

You Cannot Make a Silk Purse Out Of a Sow's Ear

There is nothing more tragic than someone whose dream exceeds his or her potential. For various reasons, some develop expectations about what is possible which are not in accord with reality. The taking of or the increasing of testosterone to overcome shortcomings will only make things worse. While there will probably be an improvement that improvement will not be enough to overcome a lack of talent.

30 Days?

While a lack of testosterone can be overcome in ways outlined in the previous chapter you may well wonder if testosterone replacement therapy is for you. It can be an expensive procedure that involves feeding your body with chemicals about which the average non pharmaceutical person has little knowledge. There are other alternatives that involve determined lifestyle change but which have proven to be very successful for moderate instances of testosterone reduction. If you implement the changes listed below over a thirty day period you should begin to see pronounced changes to both libido and testosterone levels. Even if success is limited, you will at least come away in a far better state of health and you can then take another look at other measures confident in the knowledge that you have eliminated all non chemical options.

CHAPTER 6:
THE THIRTY DAY CHALLENGE

Here is a list of lifestyle changes that you can make that should see your testosterone levels starting to elevate quite noticeably. Implement these for thirty days and then reassess your condition before attempting any other treatment.

1. Commence a weight training program. Here you should opt for heavy weight lifting that uses multiple muscle groups such as squatting and bench pressing. If you do not have access to weights or a gym then put together your own program including plenty of pushups and squats.

2. Do not over train. Up to one hour of intense weight lifting will see testosterone levels starting to improve but after that they can fall off rapidly and they may take up to five days to recover. If you are already on an endurance training program then drop that for the thirty day period and focus just on the weight program aiming for three to four sessions per week.

3. If you are carrying extra weight then start taking measures to reduce it. Excess weight has a huge number of health risks associated with it and lowering testosterone is one of them. You may believe that losing weight is impossible without doing endurance sport but in fact correct diet will be far

more beneficial than hours pounding the streets in your jogging suit.

4. Start to improve your diet. Abandon all ready meals and fast food and opt for much healthier whole foods.

5. Lose your fear of natural fat. Focus on a diet with moderate amounts of protein, plenty of natural fat such as that in fish, red meat and avocados and eat plenty of vegetables.

6. Stop alcohol altogether for the thirty day period. After that you can decide if you want to start drinking again in moderation but you may well find you would rather keep the testosterone levels up and the drink level down. Alcohol causes a twenty percent drop in most males and this figure goes up to fifty percent in alcoholics.

7. Smoking is bad for just about everything but you know that already. Use this as a motivation period for giving it up.

8. Drink plenty of water. This natural product is so often neglected but is so very important. It is not just a matter of keeping your body hydrated, you will also need to flush away the toxins generated by an unhealthy life style.

9. Make up a drink of vegetable juice from green vegetables and include a glass of that once or twice a day in your hydration plans.

10. Green vegetable are great for raising you nutrient level but broccoli, cabbage and spinach are all particularly good for testosterone elevation.

11. Garlic. This is such a wonder plant that I am surprised it is so underutilized. It contains high levels of Allicin, which is great for testosterone.

12. Take in high saturated fat by eating olive oil and cooking with coconut oil. Fat is full of nutrients and an excellent booster so don't be put off by all the myths you have heard about its effects on your weight.

13. Include raw dairy in your diet with things such as goats milk and plain full fat yoghurts.

14. Cut out sugar altogether if possible. Sugar causes a huge spike in adrenalin production and is turned to body fat quicker than anything else we eat. It contributes to raised blood pressure and type 2 diabetes, both of which are contributors to low testosterone levels. Never touch fizzy drinks and be aware that alcohol is always high in sugar.

15. Practice intermittent fasting. This has been practiced for thousands of years. You do not need to starve yourself and if you simply cram your eating into a sixteen hour window you will be allowing your body some time off to fully digest and rid its self of toxins. You can do this by simply skipping breakfast. There are dozens of other fasting regimes and I am not suggesting anything that goes beyond twenty four hours but you should definitely educate yourself as to the options here. Fasting has been shown to raise testosterone by up to 400 percent.

16. Fish oil tablets will raise your intake of vital omega three oils.

17. Ginseng is a naturally occurring plant product with testosterone raising benefits.

18. Get plenty of sunshine. You should aim at trying to be in the open air for at least an hour per day

19. If there is no sun or getting outdoors clashes with your commitments then take at least 5000 IUs of vitamin D3 per day.

20. Zinc is one substance that is often found to be deficient in men with low testosterone levels. You can take a zinc supplement. If you do choose this option then include vitamin B6 or magnesium as they both assist in the absorption of zinc.

21. Sleep is incredibly important but an often neglected area of healthy lifestyle management. Don't drink for three hours before going to sleep and sleep in a dark room. If possible do not surf the net or work on the computer in the last few

hours before going to sleep as this has been shown to make sleeping difficult.

22. Sleep in a cool room and wear cool loose fitting clothing. Your testes are in a sack rather than deep in your body because they prefer a cooler environment. Try to provide that. If possible sleep on your back or side.

23. To further moderate ideal conditions for testosterone production take cold or at least tepid showers.

24. Stress is your big enemy at the moment. Stress does immense damage to our health and its effect on our testosterone levels should not really come as surprise. Often we are stressed without even realizing it so take counter measures. Meditation is one proven technique. There are dozens of different options available here that don't involve you becoming some sort of swami. Investigate all the different methods and choose one that you can do in about ten minutes when you first get up in the morning.

25. If meditation is not your thing then consider yoga. The internet offers a vast array of beginner courses that cost nothing and which you can do in the privacy of your own home without even having to wear a caftan.

26. If both meditating and yoga are pushing you out of your comfort zone then try some plain old country walking. This is not to be looked at as a major physical work out, simply a way to let your brain decompress a little.

27. Lower your blood pressure. Well this is one that is essential for testosterone but if you have been following all of the steps above you are taking all the non medical interventions you can already so you can cross it off the list. Be aware, though, of its effects and be sure to have yours tested at your next medical visit.

28. Spend some times with friends. Laugh a little and live a little. Few things are better for de-stressing and relaxation than time spent enjoying in good company.

29. Get some sexual exercise! I know you were probably expecting you would be advised to abstain during this thirty day turnaround. In fact, sex is really good for raising endorphin levels which stimulate testosterone so if you can get it then go for it.

30. Be kind to yourself (and others). Don't go beating yourself up and raising your stress levels over this problem. Life is good. Focus on all that is positive and deliberately let go of all those mental thoughts that are polluting your mind.

So there you have it. You might be thinking this is all pretty basic but so much of being healthy is and yet how often we forget. Nature has a strange way of providing all our most basic needs and yet so often we push her aside in favor of pharmaceutical solutions thrust at us by billion dollar companies who want to get their hands into our pockets. Remember this: "Nature itself is the best physician." Hippocrates.

Final Reminder

Any decision to alter your testosterone levels through medication should only be made after consultation with medical professionals and only after thorough testing has shown your testosterone levels to be down. Be realistic in what you expect to achieve and remember that possession of testosterone is illegal unless there is a doctor's prescription.

CONCLUSION

Testosterone is the hormone responsible for masculinity and it has profound effects if the levels of it in the body are adjusted. Whilst there are chemical options for making adjustments the decision to do this should be carefully thought through and discussed with a doctor.

There are, however, plenty of ways that we can raise our testosterone levels by making healthy lifestyle changes. These bring with them the added benefit of improving your overall health, both mental and physical at the same time.

Testosterone not only affects our libido but also impacts on other areas of our lives and overall health so it is wise and understandable that we want to keep it at optimal levels. The main obstacle we need to overcome is the belief that we are helpless to make positive changes on our own. It is my belief and my experience that the suggestions offered in this book will negate the need for medical intervention.

You have nothing to lose and everything to gain so try it for thirty days and when you do so then do it whole heartedly. In just one month you have the potential to transform your life and recapture your masculinity

Thank you for downloading this book. If you enjoyed this book, then please kindly leave a review on Amazon. It would be greatly appreciated!

Thank you and good luck!

www.ingramcontent.com/pod-product-compliance
Lightning Source LLC
Chambersburg PA
CBHW071319280526
45788CB00004B/1950